Diabetic Chef

Mouthwatering Recipes to Help Control Your Blood Sugar

By

Dr. Rebecca T. Luna

Table of Contents

CHAPTER SEVEN
Beverages
A Healthy Green Smoothie Loaded with Kale and Cherries
You will need the following items to make this healthy green smoothie:
Tea with fresh mint and lemon juice served over ice.
The following ingredients are required to prepare this iced tea:
Hot Chocolate Without Added Sugar
The following ingredients are required to produce sugar-free hot chocolate:
Sparkling Water Served with a Selection of Fresh Fruit
In order to make sparkling water with fresh fruit, you will need the following ingredients:

CONCLUSION

Those with diabetes now have access to additional services and information.

INTRODUCTION

Millions of individuals throughout the world suffer from a chronic illness known as diabetes. It happens when the body is unable to effectively manufacture or utilize insulin, which results in elevated blood glucose levels. Diabetes can cause major health issues like heart disease, renal failure, and blindness if it is not properly treated. Nonetheless, many with diabetes can live healthy, productive lives with the right care.

Diet is one of the most crucial components of diabetes control. Making wise and nutritious eating decisions is essential since what we eat has a big impact on our blood sugar levels. Sadly, many diabetics have trouble planning their meals and feel they must give up their favorite foods in order to maintain their health.

The **"Diabetic Chef: Mouthwatering Recipes to Help Control Your Blood Sugar"** book comes into play here. This book is an invaluable tool for diabetics who wish to eat delectable, healthful, and simple meals without having their blood sugar levels rise.

Each of the book's several parts has recipes that have been specifically created to satisfy the nutritional requirements of those who have diabetes. The dishes are created to be low in sugar, processed carbs, and harmful fats and employ fresh, whole foods. Each dish also provides nutrition information, such as the number of calories and carbohydrates in each serving, so you can simply keep track of your intake and make wise decisions.

One of the most pervasive myths regarding diabetes is that those who have it must adhere to a bland, limited diet. The opposite is true, as you can see. You'll learn from "The Diabetic Chef" that eating well can be enjoyable and rewarding. Recipes for breakfast, nibbles, entrées, sides, desserts, and beverages may all be found here. They are all delicious and nutritious.

You can discover dishes like oatmeal with berries and almonds, spinach and feta omelet, sweet potato hash with eggs, and Greek yogurt parfaits with granola and berries, for instance, in the breakfast section. With the energy and nutrients you need to take on your everyday tasks, these meals are a terrific way to start your day off right.

Recipes like hummus with veggies, guacamole with baked tortilla chips, Caprese skewers, and smoky roasted chickpeas can all be found in the appetizers and snacks area. These meals are ideal for offering at gatherings or as daytime snacks.

You can find recipes like grilled fish with lemon and dill, turkey chili with beans, quinoa-stuffed peppers, and baked chicken parmesan in the section devoted to main meals. These dishes are not only mouth watering but also simple to prepare and loaded with nutritious components that won't cause blood sugar levels to increase. In the area devoted to sides are dishes like steamed broccoli with lemon and garlic,

quinoa pilaf with vegetables, roasted sweet
potatoes with cinnamon, and roasted
Brussels sprouts with garlic and parmesan.
These meals are a fantastic way to mix up
your meals and make sure you're getting
all the nutrients you require.
You can find recipes for chocolate
avocado pudding, berry crisp with an oat
topping, cinnamon apple chips, and
chocolate chip cookies made with almond
flour in the desert area. You may satisfy
your sweet taste with these delicacies
without worrying about raising your blood
sugar levels.
Recipes for green smoothies with kale and
berries, iced tea with lemon and fresh
mint, sugar-free hot chocolate, and
sparkling water with fresh fruit are all
found in the beverage area. Without the

added sugars that are present in many commercial beverages, these drinks are a fantastic way to remain hydrated and enjoy some tasty flavors.

In addition to the recipes, "The Diabetic Chef" offers advice on how to prepare food and manage diabetes. You'll discover how to regulate your portion sizes, interpret nutrition facts, and make healthy substitutes in your go-to recipes. Also, there are sources providing more data.

CHAPTER ONE

Keeping Blood Sugar Levels Stable Is Crucial For Persons With Diabetes.

Diabetics must pay close attention to their blood sugar levels. The eyes, kidneys, nerves, and blood arteries are all susceptible to injury from high blood sugar levels. Chronic exposure to this hazard increases the risk of developing cardiovascular disease, stroke, kidney failure, and vision loss.

The good news is that diabetics can greatly lessen their likelihood of having these issues by keeping their blood sugar levels under control. Medication, physical activity, and dietary changes are all

effective means of controlling blood sugar levels.

Controlling blood sugar levels relies heavily on dietary choices. Blood sugar levels rise after a meal because glucose, a byproduct of carbohydrate digestion, has entered the bloodstream. If a person has diabetes, their body's ability to regulate their blood sugar levels may be impaired. To control blood sugar, it's important to eat a healthy, balanced diet that's low in sugar, refined carbohydrates, and bad fats. To achieve this goal, you should stay away from sweetened beverages, processed foods, and unhealthy snack items. Diabetics should instead prioritize consuming unprocessed meals that are abundant in fiber, protein, and healthy fats.

Those with diabetes should watch their portion sizes in addition to choosing appropriate meal choices. Blood sugar levels can rise dangerously quickly after a meal, so it's vital to watch what you eat and stop when you're full rather than full. Timing of dietary interventions for blood sugar management is also crucial. Maintaining stable blood sugar levels throughout the day is facilitated by eating at regular intervals. It's also helpful to maintain steady blood sugar levels by eating a combination of carbs, protein, and healthy fats at each meal.

Regular blood sugar monitoring is also essential for those with diabetes. They can then use this information to make appropriate dietary and medicinal changes. A blood glucose meter is a tiny instrument used to determine the concentration of glucose in a blood sample.

People with diabetes should work closely with their healthcare team to build an individualized treatment strategy that includes medication, exercise, and food in addition to monitoring blood sugar levels. Considering criteria such as age, weight, exercise level, and medication regimen will help you craft a plan that works best for each person.

Medication for the control of blood sugar levels is sometimes necessary for patients with diabetes. Insulin, a hormone that aids in controlling blood sugar levels, is just one of many medications available. Both injections and insulin pumps are available for people with diabetes.

Doing regular exercise is also crucial for controlling blood sugar. Blood sugar levels can be lowered thanks to the usage of glucose as an energy source by working muscles during exercise. Insulin sensitivity can be increased with regular exercise, making it easier for the body to utilize insulin.

Those with diabetes should proceed with caution when beginning an exercise routine. Each individual's healthcare team is the best resource for helping them create a personalized, safe, and successful fitness plan that accounts for their unique needs and medical history. As a corollary, it is crucial to check blood sugar levels before, during, and after exercise to make sure they remain within a healthy range.

The bottom line is that patients with diabetes must pay close attention to their blood sugar levels. People with diabetes can dramatically lower their chance of developing serious health consequences by choosing appropriate eating choices, monitoring blood sugar levels, working closely with their healthcare team, and including exercise in their everyday lives. Those with diabetes should take an active role in controlling their illness and look for information and help when they need it. People with diabetes can live normal, productive lives if they have access to the care they need.

How eat You eat can alter your blood sugar

People with diabetes can greatly influence their blood sugar levels by changing their diet. Digesting carbohydrates results in the release of glucose into the bloodstream, which in turn causes an increase in blood sugar levels. People with diabetes need to pay special attention to the kinds and quantities of carbs they eat.
Carbohydrates are ranked on the glycemic index (GI) according to how rapidly they are broken down into glucose and absorbed by the body. Blood sugar levels can rise quickly after consuming high-GI foods like white bread, white rice, and sugary drinks, whereas they rise more

slowly after consuming low-GI foods like whole grains, fruits, and vegetables. Diabetic diets that include plenty of fiber are also crucial. The body cannot break down fiber, thus it does not cause a jump in blood sugar levels when consumed. Instead, the sluggish absorption of other carbohydrates and increased sensations of fullness and satiety are due to the fiber's contribution to blood sugar regulation. Both protein and fat have the potential to influence glucose levels. Protein and fat do not cause an increase in blood sugar levels, but they can slow the digestion and absorption of carbohydrates. Blood sugar levels may rise more slowly after eating carbohydrates when protein and fat are also consumed at the same time.

Reducing your calorie intake and increasing your exercise are both helpful in controlling your blood sugar. Overeating raises blood sugar levels, so stop eating when you're full rather than when you're satisfied. Blood sugar levels can be maintained and spikes and crashes avoided by eating smaller, more frequent meals throughout the day.

Blood sugar can be affected by more than just the types and amounts of carbs consumed. When ingested in the absence of food, alcohol can produce a rapid rise and fall in blood sugar levels. While consuming alcohol, it is best to do it in moderation and in conjunction with a meal so as to minimize the effects on blood sugar.

Also, caffeine has been shown to influence glucose metabolism. Caffeine does not directly boost blood sugar levels, but it does promote a rise in cortisol, which can have that effect. Diabetics should check their blood sugar levels before and after drinking caffeine to assess the drug's impact on their condition.

Controlling blood sugar and lowering the risk of major health consequences can be accomplished by eating a nutritious, balanced diet that is low in sugar, refined carbs, and bad fats. Fruits, vegetables, whole grains, lean protein, and healthy fats are all examples of nutrient-dense foods that can help maintain steady blood sugar levels while providing the body with the fuel it needs to perform at its best.

People with diabetes should collaborate closely with their healthcare providers to create a specialized diet plan that meets their unique requirements and tastes.

Expert advice and assistance from a registered dietician may make a big difference in how well a diabetic manage their blood sugar levels and the quality of life they are able to lead as a result of their condition.

As a result, it's clear that diet has a major impact on how a person's blood sugar levels respond to diabetes. People with diabetes can dramatically lower their chance of developing serious health consequences by adopting good eating choices, regulating portion sizes, and paying attention to the effect of different meals and beverages on their blood sugar levels. Consult with your healthcare providers to create a diet and nutrition plan that is specific to your needs and tastes. People with diabetes can live normal, productive lives if they have access to the care they need.

Dietary and preparation advice for people with diabetes

Preparing meals for someone with diabetes may seem difficult at first, but there are several tricks and techniques that may make it much simpler and more pleasurable. Some advice on what to eat and how to cook it for diabetics:

You should eat more whole foods: which are foods that are unprocessed and as close to their natural state as possible. Fruits, veggies, whole grains, lean meats, and healthy fats all fall within this category. Whole foods are preferable for people with diabetes since they are often more nutrient-dense and less processed than processed foods.

Pay attention to portion sizes
Keep in mind that controlling one's portion size is a crucial part of maintaining healthy blood sugar levels. It is possible to limit your food intake by utilizing portion-control plates, food scales, or measuring cups and spoons to measure your food.

Choose foods with a low glycemic index (GI): The rate at which carbohydrates are metabolized and absorbed by the body is quantified using a scale called the glycemic index. Whole grains, fruits, and vegetables are examples of low GI foods since they take longer to digest and hence help control blood sugar levels.

Keep sugar and processed carbs to a minimum: as these foods can produce a rapid increase in blood sugar levels. Avoiding certain items or eating them in moderation can help prevent dangerous spikes in blood sugar and other health problems.

Use healthy cooking methods: including baking, broiling, grilling, roasting, steaming, or sautéing. These techniques allow meals to retain more of their nutritional value while also reducing the number of fats and oils that are often used during preparation.

Try to stay away from fried foods: because they typically contain a lot of harmful fats and refined carbs in addition to a lot of empty calories. In addition, they can raise blood sugar levels, making them inappropriate for diabetics.

Learn from the food labels: Labels may tell you a lot about a food's nutritional value. Look for foods that are low in sugar, saturated fat, and sodium by reading the nutrition labels.

Keep an eye out for sneaky sugars: many common foods, such as sauces, condiments, and processed foods, contain sugars that are hard to detect. Look at the food's ingredient list and pick the ones with the least amount of added sugars. Good fats, such as those found in nuts, seeds, avocados, and fatty fish, can aid with glucose regulation and general health, so be sure to include them in your diet.

Consume moderate amounts of healthy fats: If you eat a wide variety of foods, you'll have a better chance of supplying your body with the nutrients it requires. Eat a wide range of colors on the plate by eating a wide range of fruits and vegetables, nutritious grains, lean proteins, and healthy fats.

To sum up, preparing meals for someone with diabetes might be difficult, but there are ways to make it less so and even fun. People with diabetes can help regulate their blood sugar levels and lessen their risk of major health issues by selecting whole meals, paying attention to portion sizes, and being conscious of hidden sugars. Individual needs and tastes should be considered when creating a tailored nutrition plan with the help of a healthcare provider and registered dietitian. People with diabetes can live normal, productive lives with the help of appropriate care and treatment.

CHAPTER TWO

Breakfast Recipes: Yummy Dishes For Morning Meals

To get your day off to a good start, try one of these tasty and diabetes-friendly breakfast recipes:

Oatmeal with Berries and Almonds

If you're looking for a healthy and filling breakfast choice that's also good for those with diabetes, try some oatmeal topped with berries and almonds. This breakfast is great for helping control blood sugar levels since it is rich in fiber, protein, and healthy fats.

Steps

Cook steel-cut or old-fashioned rolled oats to package directions before adding berries and almonds to breakfast. Cooking the oats in unsweetened almond milk instead of water is a great way to increase the nutritional value and improve the flavor. After the oats have finished cooking, they can be topped with sliced almonds and a variety of fresh berries. To sweeten it, if you like, you may add some honey or stevia.

Oats are beneficial because they include a lot of fiber, which lowers blood sugar and makes you feel full longer. Diabetics can benefit greatly from eating berries because of their low sugar content and high antioxidant content. The high quantities of protein and healthy fats in almonds have been shown to reduce hunger and improve insulin sensitivity.

As an added bonus, this breakfast may be altered to suit any tastes or dietary needs. To that end, feel free to substitute walnuts, pecans, or even pumpkin seeds for the almonds if you like. For more protein and good fats, try stirring in some plain Greek yogurt or a dollop of nut butter.

Oatmeal with berries and almonds is a cheap, quick, and easy breakfast choice that is also healthy and delicious. Individual needs and tastes should be considered when creating a tailored nutrition plan with the help of a healthcare provider and registered dietitian. Oatmeal with berries and almonds is just one example of a healthy and delicious meal that people with diabetes may have on a daily basis with proper preparation and planning.

Omelet with Feta Cheese and Spinach

Those with diabetes might benefit greatly from the nutritious and healthy spinach and feta omelet. This breakfast is a great way to start the day because of its protein, healthy fats, and fiber content.

Steps

First, in a separate bowl, beat together the eggs, salt, and pepper to produce the omelet's base. Put a tablespoon of oil or cooking spray into a pan and heat it over medium heat. Cook the chopped spinach for two to three minutes in a heated pan until it wilts. Sprinkle the spinach with the egg mixture, and heat for two to three minutes, or until the egg mixture is set around the edges. Crumble some feta cheese and sprinkle it on one side of the omelet. Fold the other side over so that the cheese is hidden within. Keep it in the oven for another minute or two until the cheese is melted and the eggs are set. Eggs are a great food choice because they include a lot of protein, which helps control hunger and satiety. Diabetics can benefit greatly from eating spinach because of its low-calorie count and high fiber, vitamin, and mineral content. Feta cheese lends a delightful tangy flavor to the omelet while also being lower in fat and calories than many other slices of cheese.

As an added bonus, this breakfast may be altered to suit any tastes or dietary needs. Vegetables like mushrooms and bell peppers, as well as different cheeses like cheddar and goat cheese, can be substituted for feta.

A spinach and feta omelet is a quick and easy breakfast choice that is not only tasty but also inexpensive and healthful. Individual needs and tastes should be considered when creating a tailored nutrition plan with the help of a healthcare provider and registered dietitian. Spinach and feta omelets are just one example of the delicious and nutritious meals that people with diabetes, with the help of the correct information and services, may enjoy every day.

Custardy Eggs with Sweet Potato Hash

Those with diabetes can benefit greatly from the combination of sweet potato hash and eggs as part of their morning meal. This breakfast is a good choice for helping to control your blood sugar levels because of its high fiber, protein, and vitamin content.

Steps

Have a sweet potato peeled and diced into little cubes to use in your egg hash. One tablespoon of oil or cooking spray, with a nonstick pan heated over medium heat, will do the trick. Add the sweet potato to the hot pan and simmer for 10 to 12 minutes, stirring periodically, until

cooked. Cook the onion, bell pepper, and garlic for about 7 minutes, or until the vegetables are tender. Separate two eggs and scatter them over the vegetables before covering the pan. Continue cooking for another two to three minutes, or until the eggs reach the doneness you choose. Vitamin A, found in abundance in sweet potatoes, is beneficial for maintaining healthy blood sugar levels and protecting the eyes from disease. Vegetables like onions and bell peppers are beneficial for persons with diabetes since they are low in calories and high in fiber and antioxidants. Eggs are a great way to get your daily dose of protein and healthy fats, both of which are important for maintaining good blood sugar levels and feeling full and satisfied.

This breakfast can also be modified to suit certain tastes and nutritional needs. Other veggies, such as mushrooms or zucchini, can be added, and the sweet potato can be replaced with butternut squash or normal potatoes. Hash can be seasoned with your favorite spices to enhance its flavor.

A breakfast of sweet potato hash with eggs is not only delicious and healthy but also quick and easy to prepare. A person's unique nutritional requirements and tastes are best met through collaboration between themselves and a healthcare provider, such as a certified dietitian. People with diabetes can still eat tasty and healthy meals like sweet potato hash with eggs every day if they have access to the correct information and services.

Greek Yogurt Parfait with Granola and Berries

A diabetic-friendly and tasty breakfast option is a Greek yogurt parfait with granola and berries. This breakfast is a great way to start the day because of the protein, fiber, and antioxidants it contains. Plain Greek yogurt, fresh berries, and granola are layered in a glass or bowl to produce a Greek yogurt parfait. Strawberries, blueberries, and raspberries work as well. Diabetics should read the nutrition label to make sure the granola they purchase is low in added sugars and rich in fiber.

Greek yogurt's high protein content makes it an ideal snack for controlling your blood sugar and feeling satisfied after eating

less. It's high in probiotics and has little carbs, both of which are beneficial to digestive health. Berries are a fantastic option for those with diabetes due to their low-calorie count, high fiber content, and a wide array of beneficial antioxidants. Since granola is packed with fiber and healthy fats, it can also include a lot of added sugars, so it's vital to pick a low-sugar kind.

This breakfast can also be modified to suit certain tastes and nutritional needs. If you're lactose sensitive or vegan, for instance, you can substitute non-dairy yogurt like soy or almond milk yogurt. To vary the texture and flavor, you can sprinkle on some nuts or seeds.

Greek yogurt parfait with granola and berries is not only a tasty and healthy breakfast option but also one that can be

prepared in advance and eaten on the go. Layer the ingredients in a mason jar or other portable container, and store them in the fridge until ready to consume. A person's unique nutritional requirements and tastes are best met through collaboration between themselves and a healthcare provider, such as a certified dietitian. Greek yogurt parfait with granola and berries is just one example of a healthy and tasty meal that individuals with diabetes may enjoy every day with the appropriate information and preparation.

CHAPTER THREE

Appetizers and Snacks

It can be hard to find appetizers and snacks that are good for people with diabetes, but there are plenty of healthy and tasty options. These little bites are great for snacking between meals or for serving at parties or other gatherings. Here are some ideas for starters and snacks that are good for people with diabetes:

Hummus with Veggies

People with diabetes can eat hummus with vegetables as an appetizer or snack because it is tasty and healthy.

Hummus is a smooth plunge produced using crushed chickpeas, tahini, lemon juice, and garlic

It is a great source of protein, fiber, and healthy fats. Carrots, cucumbers, and bell peppers are all vegetables that are low in calories and carbs and high in vitamins, minerals, and antioxidants.

Steps

Start by making the hummus. Then add the vegetables. Drain and rinse a can of chickpeas, then add them, tahini, lemon juice, garlic, and a little olive oil to a food processor. Blend until smooth and creamy, adding a splash of water if necessary to get the consistency you want. Salt and pepper can be added to taste.

Next, wash the vegetables and cut them into pieces that are easy to eat. You could use carrots, cucumbers, or bell peppers, but you can use any vegetable you like. Put the vegetables in a bowl or on a platter and serve them with the hummus.

This appetizer or snack is not only tasty but also full of nutrients that can help support your health and well-being as a whole. Chickpeas are a good source of protein and fiber, both of which can help control blood sugar levels and make you feel full. They also have a lot of vitamins and minerals, like folate, iron, and magnesium. Tahini is a paste made from ground sesame seeds. It is a good source of healthy fats, protein, and calcium. Garlic is a natural anti-inflammatory and antioxidant, and it has been shown to have many health benefits, such as lowering blood pressure and cholesterol levels. Vegetables are an important part of a healthy diet, and they can help prevent diseases like diabetes, heart disease, and cancer. They don't have many calories or carbs, but they have a lot of fiber, vitamins, minerals, and antioxidants. Adding vegetables to your meals and snacks is a simple way to get more nutrients and help your health stay at its best.

Besides being healthy and good for you, hummus with vegetables is also easy to change up to suit your tastes and dietary needs. For more flavor, you can add cumin, paprika, or parsley, among other herbs and spices, to the hummus. You can also add variety by using vegetables that aren't usually used, like radishes, jicama, or sugar snap peas. If you can't have dairy or are vegan, you can use hummus instead of ranch or blue cheese as a creamy dip for raw vegetables if you can't have dairy. Overall, hummus with vegetables is a simple and tasty way for people with diabetes to start a meal or snack. It's easy to make, you can change it up, and it's full of nutrients that can help your health and

well-being as a whole. Adding this dish to your meals and snacks is a great way to make them more interesting, tasty, and healthy.

Guacamole served with baked tortilla chips

Guacamole with baked tortilla chips is a healthy snack that people with diabetes will love. Guacamole is a dip made from

mashed avocado, lime juice, cilantro, and other spices. It is full of healthy fats, fiber, and vitamins that are good for your heart. Baked tortilla chips are a great source of complex carbohydrates and fiber, and they have less fat and calories than fried chips.

Steps

To make guacamole with baked tortilla chips, first, make the guacamole. Cut a ripe avocado in half, take out the pit, and scoop the flesh into a bowl. Mix the chopped tomato, red onion, cilantro, lime juice, and salt to taste the mashed avocado. Mix together well.

Next, turn the oven on and heat it to 350 degrees F. Make wedges out of corn tortillas and put them on a baking sheet. Use cooking spray and a pinch of salt to

season. Bake for 8 to 10 minutes, or until golden brown and crispy.

For a healthy and filling snack, serve the guacamole with the baked tortilla chips. This dish is not only tasty, but it is also full of nutrients that can help your health and well-being as a whole. Avocado has a

lot of monounsaturated fats, which can help reduce inflammation and improve cholesterol levels. It also has a lot of fiber, which can help keep blood sugar levels steady and make you feel full. Tomatoes are a good source of vitamin C and antioxidants, which can help protect against cell damage and disease. Red onions are a good source of fiber and flavonoids, which can help reduce inflammation and make the heart healthier. Traditional fried tortilla chips are often high in saturated and trans fats, but baked tortilla chips are a healthier alternative. They are made with whole-grain corn tortillas, which are a good source of complex carbohydrates and fiber. If you bake the chips instead of frying them, they have less fat and are a better choice for people with diabetes.

Guacamole with baked tortilla chips is not only healthy and nutritious, but it is also easy to change up based on personal tastes and dietary restrictions. You can add things like jalapeno peppers, garlic, or black beans to the guacamole to make it taste better and be healthier. People with celiac disease or high blood pressure can also use tortilla chips that don't have gluten or a lot of salt.

Overall, guacamole with baked tortilla chips is a good snack for people with diabetes that is both tasty and healthy. It's easy to make, you can change it up, and it's full of nutrients that can help your health and well-being as a whole. Adding this dish to your diet is a great way to make your snacks more interesting, tasty, and healthy.

Caprese skewers

Caprese skewers are a great appetizer for people with diabetes because they are easy to make and taste great. Fresh mozzarella, cherry tomatoes, and basil leaves are used to make these, and they are a good source of protein, fiber, and antioxidants.

Steps

To make caprese skewers, cut the cherry tomatoes in half and cut the fresh mozzarella into small cubes. Then, take a

skewer and put half of a cherry tomato, a basil leaf, and a cube of fresh mozzarella on it.
Continue until all the ingredients have been utilized.

Once the skewers are put together, drizzle them with olive oil and balsamic vinegar and add salt and pepper to taste. You can also put fresh basil leaves on top to make them look and taste better.

Caprese skewers are not only tasty, but they are also full of nutrients that can help improve your health and well-being as a whole. Cherry tomatoes are a good source of vitamin C and antioxidants, which can help protect cells from damage and disease. Fresh mozzarella is a good source of protein and calcium, which are important for building and keeping strong bones and muscles. The leaves of basil are a good source of vitamins A and K, which can help keep your immune system healthy and your bones strong.

Caprese skewers are not only healthy, but they are also a great way to spice up your appetizers and give them more variety. You can change them to fit your tastes and any dietary restrictions. For example, you can add flavor and texture by using different kinds of cheese, like feta or goat cheese. You can also add other healthy and tasty ingredients, such as olives or roasted red peppers.

Overall, Caprese skewers are a healthy and tasty way for people with diabetes to start a meal. They are easy to make, can be changed to fit your needs, and are full of nutrients that can help your health and well-being as a whole. Adding this dish to your diet is a great way to make your meals more interesting, tasty, and healthy

Chickpeas roasted with spices

Spicy roasted chickpeas are a great snack for people with diabetes because they are healthy and tasty. Chickpeas are a great source of fiber, protein, and many important vitamins and minerals. They also have a low glycemic index, which means they don't cause blood sugar levels to rise quickly. Roasting them with spices makes them taste better and gives them more nutrients.

Steps

Start by setting your oven to 400°F before you put the chickpeas in. Drain, rinse, and pat dry a can of chickpeas with a paper towel. In a bowl, mix the chickpeas with 1 tablespoon of olive oil, 1 teaspoon of smoked paprika, 1/2 teaspoon of garlic powder, and a pinch of salt and black pepper. Spread the chickpeas out on a baking sheet and roast them for 20 to 25 minutes, stirring them every now and then, until they are golden brown and crispy. Spicy roasted chickpeas are a great alternative to snacks like potato chips and pretzels that are high in carbs and fat. They are easy to make, can be changed to suit your tastes, and can be seasoned with many different spices. They are also a great addition to salads and soups, and they can be used to add more protein to the trail mix.

CHAPTER FOUR

Main Dishes

Dishes that are traditionally considered to be the centerpieces of a dinner also play a significant part for diabetics in terms of controlling their blood sugar levels. While putting together a meal, it's crucial to choose foods that are low in carbohydrates, high in fiber and protein, and rich in vitamins and minerals. This will ensure that you get the most out of your meal. The following are some recipes for mouthwatering main dishes that are suitable for individuals who have diabetes:

Grilled Salmon with Asparagus and Lemon

Salmon that has been grilled is an excellent main course option because it is high in protein and has a good amount of omega-3 fatty acids. The vegetable asparagus has a relatively low carbohydrate content and a high concentration of fiber, vitamin C, and mineral content.

Steps

To begin preparing this meal, begin by marinating the salmon for half an hour in a mixture of lemon juice, olive oil, garlic, and seasonings such as salt and pepper. Grill the salmon for five to six minutes on each side, or until it reaches an internal temperature of 145 degrees Fahrenheit. As the salmon is being grilled, prepare the asparagus by tossing it with olive oil, seasoning it with salt and pepper, and then roasting it in the oven for 10 to 12 minutes. To enhance the flavor of the salmon and asparagus, serve them with wedges of lemon.

Chicken and Vegetable Stir-Fry

A stir-fry is a meal that can be prepared quickly and easily, and it can be adapted to incorporate a wide variety of low-carbohydrate vegetables as well as lean proteins.

Steps

To begin preparing this meal, begin by marinating chicken breasts for half an hour in a marinade that includes soy sauce, ginger, garlic, and sesame oil. Put one tablespoon of oil into a wok or a large skillet and then place it over high heat. Stir fry the chicken for

around four to five minutes, or until it reaches an internal temperature of 165 degrees. Stir-frying will continue for an additional three to four minutes with the addition of cut veggies such as bell peppers, broccoli, and snap peas. Salt, pepper, and additional soy sauce should be added based on personal preference. To increase the amount of fiber and nutrients in the dish, serve it with quinoa or brown rice.

Spaghetti Squash with Turkey Meatballs

Meatballs and Parmesan Garlic Bread Because it is lower in carbohydrates and higher in fiber than typical pasta, spaghetti squash makes for an excellent substitute for that food.

Steps

To begin preparing this recipe, begin by roasting a spaghetti squash in the oven for thirty to forty
minutes, or until it reaches the desired level of tenderness. While the squash is in the oven, prepare the meatballs by combining the ground turkey with the breadcrumbs, egg, parsley, garlic, and seasonings of your choice. In a large

skillet set over medium heat, brown the meatballs in the pan. After adding the crushed tomatoes, continue to boil for another 10 to 15 minutes. After the spaghetti squash has been cooked, you can produce "noodles" by scraping the flesh of the squash with a fork. The turkey meatballs and tomato sauce should be served on top of the spaghetti squash before serving.

Pork Tenderloin on the Barbecue, Accompanied by Roasted Vegetables

The pork tenderloin is a cut of meat that is strong in protein and low in carbs, in addition to being a tasty and lean cut of meat.

Steps

To begin preparing this dish, begin by marinating the pork for half an hour in a combination consisting of olive oil, garlic, rosemary, salt, and pepper. Cook the pork on the grill for 4-5 minutes per side, or until it reaches an internal temperature of 145 degrees Fahrenheit. As the pork is being grilled, roast a variety of vegetables including sweet potatoes, Brussels sprouts, and carrots in the oven for 20 to 25 minutes with olive oil, salt, and pepper. For a supper that is both satiating and beneficial to your health, serve the grilled pork with veggies that have been roasted.

Cauliflower fried rice with shrimp

If you're looking for a tasty and nutritious alternative to regular fried rice, try making cauliflower fried rice with shrimp instead. Cauliflower, which has been finely diced, serves as the base of this dish rather than rice. Cauliflower has a lower carbohydrate content and a higher fiber content than rice. The incorporation of shrimp results in an increase in available protein, and the use of vegetables such as carrots, peas, and green onions enhance both the flavor and the nutritional value of the dish.

Steps

To begin preparing this dish, begin by reducing the size of the cauliflower florets to a consistency similar to that of rice grains by pulsing them in a food processor. Then, in a big skillet, sauté the cauliflower with garlic and ginger until it reaches the desired tenderness. The eggs should be scrambled until they are fully cooked, so push the cauliflower to one side of the pan and add the beaten eggs to the other.

The next step is to add shrimp that has been cooked together with a sauce made of soy sauce, sesame oil, and rice vinegar to the skillet. After stirring them in, continue cooking the vegetables until they are completely warmed through. To serve, bring to a boil and drizzle with additional soy sauce or hot sauce, if preferred.

Those who are adhering to a ketogenic diet or a low-carbohydrate diet, in addition to those who are seeking a savory main dish that is also nutritious, should consider selecting this dish as an alternative. Including cauliflower and other vegetables in your diet is an excellent method to increase your intake of veggies, which is important because vegetables supply a wide range of vitamins and minerals.

CHAPTER FIVE

Side Dishes

The addition of taste, nutrition, and variety to any meal is easily accomplished through the use of side dishes. When it comes to the control of blood sugar levels for persons who have diabetes, selecting the appropriate side dishes might be of the utmost importance. These scrumptious side dishes are not only delicious but also appropriate for diabetics:

Brussel Brussels Sprouts with Garlic and Parmesan

A side dish that is not only easy to make but also flavorful and nutritious, roasted Brussels sprouts with garlic and Parmesan are a wonderful option. Brussels sprouts are an excellent source of fiber, vitamin C, and vitamin K, and the addition of garlic and Parmesan gives the dish a flavor that is both robust and delicious.

Steps

Begin by bringing your oven up to a temperature (of 400 degrees Fahrenheit) so that you may roast the Brussels sprouts with garlic and Parmesan. Remove the tough ends of the Brussels sprouts and cut them in half lengthwise. Next, place the

Brussels sprouts in a bowl and add some olive oil, minced garlic, salt, and pepper. Place the Brussels sprouts in a single layer on a baking sheet, and then roast them in the oven for 20 to 25 minutes, stirring once or twice, until they are soft and have developed a browned exterior.

When the Brussels sprouts are ready, remove them from the oven, place them in a bowl, and then sprinkle them with grated Parmesan cheese. The roasted Brussels sprouts should be served hot as a side dish along with your preferred main entrée. This recipe is a wonderful method to increase the number of vegetables you consume on a daily basis and to add some diversity to the meals you eat.

Pilaf with Quinoa and Vegetables to Serve

A nutrient-dense and satiating side dish, quinoa pilaf with veggies is the kind of dish that works well for any event. While veggies not only contribute a variety of nutrients but also color and flavor to the dish, quinoa is a complete protein and a rich source of fiber, vitamins, and minerals.

Steps

In order to make quinoa pilaf with vegetables, you need to begin by rinsing the quinoa in a colander with a fine-mesh screen to remove any bitterness. Bring the quinoa, liquid (either water or broth), and

a pinch of salt to a boil in a saucepan. Once the liquid is absorbed and the quinoa is soft, turn the heat down to low, cover the saucepan, and continue to simmer the quinoa for 15–20 minutes.

When the quinoa is cooking, you can get started on preparing the vegetables. You are free to use whichever mix of vegetables strikes your fancy, such as carrots, bell peppers, zucchini, and onions. You should cut the vegetables up into bite-sized pieces and then sauté them in a pan with some olive oil until they are soft and have a faint browning on them.

Once the quinoa and the vegetables are done cooking, mix them in a big bowl and toss them together to integrate the flavors. Salt, pepper, and any other herbs and spices that you enjoy, such as parsley, basil, or thyme, should be used to season

the quinoa pilaf. You may also add some nuts or seeds, such as almonds or sunflower seeds, for an extra crunch as well as some additional nutrients.

You can have the quinoa pilaf with vegetables as a side dish with grilled chicken or fish, or you can have it on its own as a main dish for vegetarians. This recipe is a wonderful method to increase the number of nutritious grains and veggies that you consume on a daily basis, as well as to add some variety to the meals that you eat.

Yummy Sweet Potatoes with Cinnamon That Have Been Roasted

A tasty and nutritious side dish that is ideal for the fall and winter months is

roasted sweet potatoes spiced with cinnamon. Cinnamon provides the dish with a flavor that is both warm and spicy, while sweet potatoes are an excellent source of fiber, vitamins, and minerals.

Steps

First things first, preheat the oven to 400 degrees Fahrenheit so you may create roasted sweet potatoes with cinnamon. After being peeled and diced into bite-sized pieces, the sweet potatoes should be tossed in a bowl with some olive oil, ground cinnamon, salt, and pepper. Place the sweet potatoes in a single layer on a baking sheet, and then roast them in the oven for 20 to 25 minutes, stirring once or twice, until they

are cooked and have developed a golden brown color.
After the sweet potatoes have finished cooking, place them in a serving dish and

top them with a few additional pinches of ground cinnamon. Serve the roasted sweet potatoes hot as a side dish with your favorite main course. This recipe is a wonderful method to increase the number of vegetables you consume on a daily basis and to add some diversity to the meals you eat. It's also a fantastic alternative to typical sweet potato meals that are filled with sugar and butter.

Steamed Broccoli with Lemon and Garlic

Steamed broccoli with lemon and garlic is a healthful and savory side dish that is

quick and easy to prepare. Broccoli is a nutritious vegetable that is rich in vitamins and minerals, while lemon and garlic provide a vibrant and tangy flavor to the dish.

Steps

To cook steamed broccoli with lemon and garlic, start by cleaning the broccoli and cutting it into bite-sized florets. Put the broccoli in a steamer basket over a saucepan of boiling water and steam it for 5-7 minutes, until it is soft but still a little crunchy.

When the broccoli is steaming, prepare the lemon and garlic sauce. Mince a few cloves of garlic and zest a lemon, then put them in a small bowl with some lemon juice, olive oil, salt, and pepper. Mix the

ingredients together until they are fully blended.

When the broccoli is done, transfer it to a serving dish and pour the lemon and garlic sauce over it. Toss the broccoli in the sauce to coat it evenly. Garnish the dish with some chopped parsley or grated Parmesan cheese, if preferred.

Steamed broccoli with lemon and garlic is a terrific side dish to offer with grilled chicken, fish, or tofu. It's also an excellent way to include extra vegetables in your diet and get a boost of vitamins and minerals. The lemon and garlic sauce lends a bright and zesty flavor to the dish that balances the earthy flavor of the broccoli.

CHAPTER SIX

Desserts

Finding appetizers and snacks that are suitable for people with diabetes can be difficult, but there are many tasty choices that are both nutritious and filling. These bite-sized treats are ideal for serving at events or parties as well as for sating hunger pangs in between meals. A few suggestions for diabetic-friendly appetizers and snacks are included below:

Avocado Chocolate Pudding

Another creamy and delightful dish that is suitable for people with diabetes is chocolate avocado pudding. Ripe avocados are blended with cocoa powder, almond milk, vanilla extract, and a sweetener of your choice, such as stevia or honey, to create this dessert.

While the cocoa powder is abundant in flavanols, which have been shown to enhance blood flow and lessen inflammation in the body, avocados are a fantastic source of fiber and healthy fats. The addition of almond milk and a sweetener can help balance the flavors and make a tasty and rich dessert that is also reduced in carbohydrates and sugar.

Steps

Ripe avocados should first be processed or blended into a smooth paste in a food processor or blender to produce chocolate avocado pudding. Add your preferred sweetener, cocoa powder, almond milk, and vanilla extract, and continue mixing until the mixture is creamy and thoroughly blended. According to your tastes, you can modify the sweetness level to taste.

Once the pudding is thoroughly combined, divide it among serving jars or bowls and chill it for at least an hour to let it set. For additional taste and texture, you can garnish the pudding with fresh berries, whipped cream, or chopped almonds.

For those with diabetes who want to indulge in something sweet and creamy

without experiencing substantial blood sugar rises, chocolate avocado pudding is a perfect alternative. Also, it is an excellent method to add fiber and healthy fats to your diet, which can help control blood sugar levels and enhance general health.

Berry Crisp with Oat Topping

A delicious and healthful dessert choice that is ideal for diabetics is berry crisp with oat topping. These berries—strawberries, raspberries, and blueberries—can be used fresh or frozen. A crumbly topping of oats, almonds, cinnamon, and your preferred sweetener, like coconut sugar or maple syrup, is then sprinkled on top.

Antioxidants and fiber, which are abundant in berries, can help control blood

sugar levels and enhance general health. Oats and almonds are added to the recipe to give complex carbohydrates and good fats that can help reduce blood sugar spikes and absorption of sugar.

Steps

Start by heating your oven to 375°F in preparation for making berry crisp with oat topping. Fill a baking dish with the berry mixture, and then set it aside. Combine oats, chopped almonds, cinnamon, and your preferred sweetener in a separate mixing dish. Sprinkle the crumbly mixture over the berry mixture in the baking dish after combining all the ingredients.

For about 30 minutes, or until the topping is golden brown and the fruit mixture is

bubbling, bake the berry crisp in the oven. When the crisp is finished baking, take it out of the oven and allow it cool before serving. For more flavor and decadence, top the crisp with a dollop of whipped cream or a scoop of vanilla ice cream.

For diabetics who wish to indulge in something sweet without jeopardizing their health, berry crisp with oat topping is a delightful and healthy dessert alternative. It is simple to prepare and may be tailored to your tastes by using the berries and sweets of your choice.

Cinnamon apple chips

A quick and delectable dessert option that is ideal for diabetics is cinnamon apple chips. Thinly sliced apples are combined with cinnamon and your preferred sweeteners, such as stevia or honey, to

make this treat. After that, the apple slices are roasted in the oven until crisp and golden.

The high fiber and nutrient content of apples can help control blood sugar levels and enhance general health. Cinnamon adds a sweet and smoky flavor that might help lower blood sugar levels and lessen sugar cravings.

Steps

Start by setting your oven to 200°F in preparation for making cinnamon apple chips.
A baking pan should be covered in parchment paper and left alone.
Your preferred apple should be cleaned and thinly sliced with the seeds and cores removed. Combine cinnamon and the

sweetener of your choice in a small mixing basin. Being sure to cover both sides, sprinkle the mixture over the apple slices.
The apple slices should be baked for about 2-3 hours, or until they are crisp and golden brown, in a layer on the baking

sheet that has been prepared. When the chips are finished baking, take them out of the oven and allow them cool before serving.

A delicious and healthy dessert choice that is simple to make and ideal for sating your sweet desire without jeopardizing your health is cinnamon apple chips. They can be eaten as a snack or as a dessert with a drizzle of honey or a dollop of Greek yogurt.

Almond flour cookies with chocolate chips

Almond flour chocolate chip cookies are a delicious and nutritious alternative to regular cookies, making them a fantastic option for those with diabetes. Protein, fiber, and healthy fats found in abundance in almond flour can help control blood sugar levels and encourage feelings of fullness.

Steps

The first step in making chocolate chip cookies with almond flour is to preheat your oven to 350°F. Almond flour, baking soda, and salt should all be combined in a sizable mixing dish. Melted butter, an egg, vanilla extract, and a sweetener of your

choice, such as honey or stevia, should be combined in a separate bowl.
After adding the wet components to the dry ones, thoroughly combine.
Add chocolate chunks or chips and combine.
Drop the dough onto a baking sheet lined with parchment using a cookie scoop or spoon.

Bake for 10 to 12 minutes, or until the edges are lightly browned.

The cookies should cool for a few minutes before being moved to a wire rack to finish cooling.

A wonderful and nutritious treat that can be enjoyed any time of the day is these cookies with chocolate chips and almond flour. Without raising your blood sugar levels, they are ideal for fulfilling your sweet tooth. Also, they are simple to

produce and may be kept for up to a week in an airtight container.

CHAPTER SEVEN

Beverages

For diabetics, the management of their blood sugar levels is significantly impacted by the beverages they consume. If you select the appropriate beverages, you can help minimize spikes in blood sugar and maintain proper hydration without adding an excessive amount of sugar or calories to your diet.

Because it does not have any sugar or calories, water is always the greatest choice for keeping yourself hydrated. The addition of a slice of cucumber, lemon, or lime can provide more taste and make the beverage more pleasurable to consume.

Warm beverages, such as green tea and unsweetened herbal tea, can also be calming and comforting to the body and mind. **The following is a list of beverages that you might want to think about.**

A Healthy Green Smoothie Loaded with Kale and Cherries

Those who have diabetes may find that drinking a green smoothie that is low in carbohydrates and nutrient-dense is an effective strategy to help them better regulate their blood sugar levels. This particular dish calls for kale and berries, both of which are low in sugar while being high in various antioxidants and other minerals.

You will need the following items to make this healthy green smoothie:

1 cup kale leaves, chopped
1/2 cup of the frozen berry mixture, blended
1/2 tiny banana
1/2 cup of almond milk that has not been sweetened
1/2 cup ice
Put all of the ingredients in a blender, and run it until the mixture is completely smooth. If the smoothie is too thick for your liking, you can adjust the consistency

by adding additional almond milk or water.

The green vegetable known as kale is an excellent source of vitamins A, C, and K,

in addition to calcium and other minerals. Berries, including blueberries, raspberries, and blackberries, are excellent sources of both fiber and antioxidants. The little amount of banana contributes a hint of sweetness without significantly elevating the level of sugar in the blood.

This green smoothie is a delicious and refreshing way to add some nutritious greens and antioxidants to your diet. It is also a terrific option for breakfast or as a snack in between meals. After ingesting this, or any other food or beverage for that matter, it is essential to pay attention to the quantity of food consumed and to check blood sugar levels.

Tea with fresh mint and lemon juice served over ice.

Iced tea flavored with fresh mint and lemon is an invigorating and savory beverage that is ideal for hot weather or any other time of year when you desire a cold beverage that satisfies your thirst. Because it does not call for any additional sugar and can assist in maintaining healthy blood sugar levels, this recipe is an excellent choice for those who suffer from diabetes.

The following ingredients are required to prepare this iced tea:

4 ounces of water

4 tea bags (black or green tea)

a quarter of a cup of fresh mint leaves
1/2 lemon, sliced
Ice cubes
The water should be brought to a boil in a large pot, at which point the heat should be turned off and the tea bags, mint leaves, and lemon slices should be added. After allowing the tea to steep for 10 to 15 minutes, take out the tea bags and strain the liquid through a sieve with a fine mesh. Let it reach room temperature before placing it in the refrigerator to chill completely.
If preferred, more mint leaves and lemon slices can be used as garnishes for the iced tea after it has been served over ice cubes. This iced tea is a tasty and nutritious alternative to sugary drinks due to the natural sweetness of the mint as well as

the acidity of the lemon. In addition, the vitamin C found in lemon and the antioxidants found in tea combine to make this beverage a nutritious powerhouse.

Hot Chocolate Without Added Sugar

Sugar-free hot chocolate is a tasty and comforting treat that can be appreciated by persons with diabetes as well as anyone wanting to limit the amount of sugar in their diet. This recipe for rich and creamy hot chocolate that won't cause your blood sugar to surge utilizes unsweetened cocoa powder as the base and a sugar replacement as the sweetener.

The following ingredients are required to produce sugar-free hot chocolate:

2 cups of almond milk, sweetened to taste (or milk of your choice)

2 teaspoons of cocoa powder that have not been sweetened

1-2 tablespoons sugar replacement (such as stevia, erythritol, or Splenda)

1/2 teaspoon vanilla extract

A little bit of salt

To make almond milk, place the milk in a small saucepan and heat it over medium heat until it starts to steam. Mix the cocoa powder, sugar replacement, vanilla extract, and salt together with a whisk until the mixture is smooth and uniform. Keep heating the mixture over the stove until it

reaches the temperature you want it at,
then pour it into mugs and serve it.
You won't feel guilty about indulging in
this sugar-free hot chocolate because it's
so delicious and will satisfy your needs for
chocolate. In addition, you have the option
of experimenting with various milk
replacements, such as cashew milk or
coconut milk or adding a pinch of
cinnamon or nutmeg for an additional
layer of taste.

Sparkling Water Served with a Selection of Fresh Fruit

Those who have diabetes or anyone else
who is trying to minimize the amount of
sugar they consume would benefit greatly

from drinking sparkling water with fresh fruit because it is both a healthy and delicious beverage option. When you combine fresh fruit with carbonated water to make this beverage, you get a naturally flavored and bubbly beverage that is not only delectable but also good for your hydration.

In order to make sparkling water with fresh fruit, you will need the following ingredients:

Dazzling water
Ice, along with freshly cut fruit (such as melons, berries, or citrus),
First, fill a glass with ice cubes, then add the necessary amount of fresh fruit, and last, stir the mixture. You can use just one kind of fruit, or you can combine other

kinds of fruits to create a more nuanced flavor. The next step is to fill the glass with sparkling water until it is completely full. After combining the fruit with the sparkling water in the drink by giving it a brief stir, you may then enjoy it. Because it is made with fresh fruit, this beverage is not only delicious but also abundant in the vitamins and antioxidants that the fruit provides. It is an excellent replacement for sugary drinks or juice, and it can be had at any time of the day. You can also try out a variety of flavor combinations in order to find the one that you like best, such as cucumber and mint, pineapple and ginger, and so on.

CONCLUSION

To summarize, maintaining an appropriate level of blood sugar control is an integral element of coping with diabetes. The good news is that it is possible to control blood sugar levels and lead a healthy, meaningful life by making the proper decisions regarding nutrition and lifestyle. Although this can be a challenge, the good news is that it is doable. The recipes contained in The **"Diabetic Chef: Mouthwatering Recipes to Help Manage Your Blood Sugar"** have been developed specifically for individuals who have diabetes, with an emphasis placed on the utilization of wholesome, nutrient-dense ingredients that will assist in maintaining stable blood sugar levels.

The recipes in this book cover every meal of the day, from breakfast to dessert, and offer a diverse array of tastes and textures to satiate any appetite. It doesn't matter if you're in the mood for a hearty omelet, a crunchy snack, or a sweet treat; whatever it is you're looking for, you're sure to discover something that not only satisfies your dietary requirements but also tastes wonderful.

In addition to the actual recipes, this book also provides helpful advice and information regarding the ways in which one's food and way of life might affect one's blood sugar levels. The readers are able to make more educated decisions about what they eat and how they prepare their meals if they get a deeper understanding of the science that underpins diabetes and how it is connected to nutrition. This book is an excellent resource for anyone who wants to regulate their blood sugar levels and improve their general health because it provides helpful tips on controlling portion sizes, planning meals, and shopping for nutritious products.

Overall, **The Diabetic Chef: Mouthwatering Recipes to Help Control Your Blood Sugar** is a book that everyone who lives with diabetes or is wanting to embrace a better lifestyle absolutely needs to have in their collection. This book is guaranteed to become a go-to resource for anyone who is trying to take control of their blood sugar levels and improve their overall health and well-being due to the fact that it contains delectable recipes, useful ideas, and directions that are simple to follow. Why hold off then? Get your kitchen in gear and start whipping up some delectable dishes so you can start reaping the benefits of a diabetes-friendly diet right away.

Those with diabetes now have access to additional services and information.

People who have diabetes have access to a wide variety of supplementary tools and informational sources that can assist in the management of their illness.

The American Diabetes Association is an excellent site that provides a plethora of information on the management of diabetes. Its information covers a variety of topics, such as the planning of meals, the management of the physical activity, and the administration of medication. They also offer information for people who are in need of aid navigating insurance and financial assistance programs and who are in need of support.

The Centers for Disease Control and Prevention (CDC), which includes information on diabetes prevention and management as well as services for healthcare providers, is yet another useful resource.

There are many online forums and support groups for people who have diabetes. These are places where people can talk about their experiences, ask questions, and get advice from others who are living with the condition. Those who are looking for support and a sense of community should check out these resources.

Last but not least, it is essential for people who have diabetes to build an individualized strategy for managing their condition through close collaboration with their healthcare team. This team should include their primary care provider,

endocrinologist, and registered dietitian. Diabetes can be managed well and complications avoided by those who get routine medical examinations and keep close tabs on their blood sugar levels.

www.ingramcontent.com/pod-product-compliance
Lightning Source LLC
Chambersburg PA
CBHW070745250726
48662CB00004B/1644